Treating

Holistically with

Cannabis:

Handcrafted Cannabis Ointments, Salves, & Tinctures

Volume 2

Learn how to create unique cannabis infused ointments, salves, and tinctures for topically treating your pain and ailments!

By Marie J. Burke

Treating Holistically with Cannabis

Handcrafted Ointments, Salves, & Tinctures Volume 2

Sunny Cabana Publishing, L.L.C.

www.sunnycabanapublishing.com

By Marie J. Burke

Published by Sunny Cabana Publishing, L.L.C.
Printed in the United States of America
Author: Marie J. Burke
13-digit ISBN: 978-1-936874-32-3
10-digit ISBN: 1936874326
First Printing

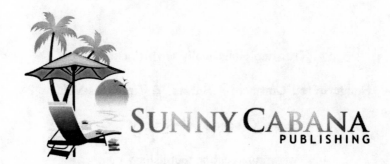

Disclaimer:
The responsibility for any adverse detoxification effects resulting from using these recipes described lies not with the author or distributors of this book. This book is not intended for medical advice just as suggestion. So please seek a doctor first in your community to get advice and consultations. Also make sure that it is legal in the state that you live!

Please enjoy these recipes with your friends and family to help support the natural healing of our bodies through the use of natural remedies.

Cannabis doesn't lead to an increased risk of lung cancer.

In 5000 years of recorded history there is not one case of lung cancer attributed to cannabis use alone.

Dr. Donald Tashkin of UCLA conducted a study in order to prove that cannabis use was linked to lung cancer.

Surprisingly, no association was found between the two, even in chronic long time users. They observed that cannabis dilates the airways, as opposed to tobacco, and is an effective treatment against asthma and emphysema.

Please use responsibly!

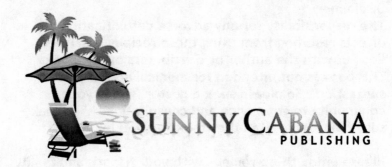

Contents

Intro

I have been a health advocate for many years now and have dedicated most of my life to eating organic, supporting local farmers, and learning all I can about the benefits of good wholesome food. I think that food or anything that you ingest or use on your body should be as natural as possible. That is why I decided to try to find out as much information that I could on the benefits of using cannabis or marijuana ointments, salves, and tinctures on the body. There is so much hype today on whether or not to use the product or even if it really helps and if it does help how does one make the wonderful treatment.

I wanted to know what questions people were asking when it came to cannabis ointments, salves, and tinctures, and if they knew the benefits or even how to prepare the product. I live in a state where the product is legalized for medicinal purposes and I started to ask questions and got answers. I wanted to share my experiences with people like myself who were not as experienced in the field of alternative natural healing and that is how this whole thing got started....

There are several different ways to prepare cannabis for either ingesting or using it topically in order to help with many ailments. It is really important to make sure that you are living in a state that cannabis is legal and that you have the appropriate doctor prescribe the correct dosage for your body type and ailment.

I will go over the benefits and diseases that can benefit from cannabis infused products and how to make cannabis salves, ointments, and tinctures. I will also go over what items you will need in the kitchen, different oils that are used in the process, and the benefit of mixing certain essential oils in your salves and ointments. Cannabis ointments, salves, and tinctures made simple and easy!

If you are hurting and you prefer to not inhale cannabis smoke into your lungs than I hope this book helps! The more you know about how to take care of yourself the better off you will be!

*Please make sure that you label all of your medicines and keep them far away from small hands. Use responsibly.

The Benefits of Topical Cannabis

Cannabis has been used for many years for a variety
of topical applications. Cannabis infused products
can be absorbed directly into the skin, joints, and
ligaments to help with many ailments. By using a

topical cannabinoid product you can reduce the side effects of ingesting or smoking cannabis to your body. When you apply a topical cannabis product you are localizing it to a specific area that is hurting, inflamed, or in pain. When you smoke or ingest cannabis your whole body feels the effects of cannabinoids, which would be used for different ailments.

Cannabis infused salves and ointments has such a wonderful benefit to people who have either a pulled muscle, skin irritation, or have arthritic joints. You can use the cannabis product right where the pain is! Plus your body does not experience the high effect from ingesting or smoking cannabis. Cannabis infused products will be the medicine of the future in all states eventually because cannabis can heal so many ailments. Why not have this wonderful product available so that everyone can use it! Cannabis salves and ointments are so versatile and help with so many different ailments it may be the only medicine that you will need!

Cannabis products are excellent for many skin infections or disorders. Here are just a few of them:

- ✓ Eczema
- ✓ Psoriasis
- ✓ Dermatitis
- ✓ Bursitis
- ✓ Cuts
- ✓ Scrapes

- ✓ Wrinkles
- ✓ Skin discolorations
- ✓ Burns (yes, even 2nd degree)
- ✓ Regenerative effects
- ✓ Antibacterial effects
- ✓ Helps with fungal diseases such as nail fungus, athletes feet, corns
- ✓ Clearing away acne
- ✓ Herpes on the lips or fever blisters
- ✓ Hemorrhoids
- ✓ Menstrual cramps
- ✓ Colds and sore throat
- ✓ Asthma
- ✓ Inflammation of the larynx

*Please note: Do not put the salves, ointments, or tinctures directly on a bleeding wound.

Cannabis oil is very good for relieving pain with such ailments like:

- ✓ Arthritic pain
- ✓ Swelling in the joints
- ✓ Muscle spasms
- ✓ Sore muscles
- ✓ Reduces nausea
- ✓ Helps with migraines
- ✓ Maybe even cancer (I have seen many instances where cannabis salves have decreased or even taken individuals skin cancers completely away)

How can one product do so much and not be legal everywhere? It's an amazing healing product that can be used daily on all of your ailments and skin disorders.

Plain and simple; what is a cannabinoid and how does it work in our body? Now I am not a scientist or a doctor but I do know the basics on how cannabinoids works with our bodies and I am sure that there is much more information out there regarding this subject and in much more detail then I will be describing but I just wanted to give you a simple review on the subject first before you scoured the world for cannabinoid information.

Cannabinoids (CBD) or THC is the main active ingredient in cannabis. CBD does not induce euphoria with topical application but does help with reducing inflammation in the body on and around the arthritic joints and reduces many antibacterial skin ailments.

Topical cannabis stimulates localized THC and CBD receptors throughout our bodies. These receptors are called CB1 and CB2 and they are both located in our bodies. CB1 is our mental receptors and CB2 is related to our immune system, which is mostly why we get sick or have skin and body disorders because our immune system is lacking something. The CBD attaches to the CB2 receptors to help with inflammation, pain, and many various skin diseases.

Topical or transdermal cannabis can be absorbed directly into the skin to the affected areas where you have pain or an ailment. Cannabis is lipophilic, which just simply means it can be dissolved in a fat soluble substance such as coconut oil, olive oil, Shea butter, etc. When the cannabis is topically infused with certain oils and creams and then used on your skin it has a pain and inflammation reducing effect on the body along with helping with many other ailments and skin disorders that you may have. Transdermal cannabis goes directly into the skin and is one of the best ways to administer medicine into your body because it is so easily absorbed. Also when you are applying the transdermal cannabis it is not absorbed into the liver or stomach so your body is getting the cannabis directly to the painful area without interruption from the stomach and liver functions. When you use transdermal cannabis you will have fewer side effects then from ingesting cannabis like no drowsiness and no upset stomach. I have also seen where patients have added topical magnesium chloride to their cannabis salves because it helps with really severe pain. Plus the essential and regular oils that you will be using in these recipes have many other great benefits for your body so it is a win~ win situation!

If you are tired of not living your life to its fullest because of pain or skin irritations then maybe you should look to other natural sources for pain relief such as cannabis infused products. Maybe you want to get rid of or reduce the amount of eczema, acne, or wrinkles you have. Well this is the product for you! It's always a good idea to keep cannabis oil or cannabis salve in your house for things like burns, antibacterial problems, or pain. This guide will show you how to simply make cannabis ointments, salves, and creams so that you can keep this wonderful medicine in your household. Just please remember that not all states allow this and check with your state legislation first before making such products! And again make sure that you label your medicine and keep out it out of reach from small hands.

Preparing Your Kitchen

To get started you will need to have a few items in your kitchen (you probably already have many of these items). By having these items you will have a much higher success rate at producing your cannabis salves or ointments. Make sure that you start with a clean area and have everything 'mise en place' (French for everything in place) so that it will make the process go smoothly. There is nothing worse than starting a project and not having the right materials. You do not want to make your life more frustrating by not having what you need and where you need it. It is just like making your favorite cookies or cake you always make sure that you have all of your ingredients before you start the process right? You want the process to be fun not stressful. By having all of your items in order you will be able to focus on the things that matter, like the consistency, the smell, and the packaging. Make sure that you block out enough time to dedicate to this process because there is nothing worse than being interrupted by the phone, computer, or people. Don't be nervous just dive in! You may even come up with your own great recipe by experimenting with the right tools and the right ingredients.

Here is a list of kitchen items that you will need in order to process and make your own cannabis tinctures, salves, ointments, and creams.

Cooking Utensils

- Coffee Grinder
- Crock Pot

- Double Boiler
- Cheese Cloth for straining the cannabis
- Nylons for straining the cannabis
- Fine Metal Strainer
- Jars with the Lids (all kinds and sizes because you may want to use smaller jars to hand out as gifts or you may just want smaller batches. You can easily find these on the internet).
- Empty Lip Balm Containers (If you want to make lip balm. You can find these on the internet.)
- Small Metal Containers (If that's what you want to store your salves in. A glass jar will work fine though.)
- Sticky Labels; to mark the date, mixture, and type of product.
- Disposable Gloves
- Measuring Cups
- Measuring Spoons
- Mixing Spoons
- Mixing Bowls
- Small Measuring Scale
- Funnels
- Coffee Filters
- Spatulas

You may find that you will use different kitchen tools but the above tools are always a good start to your adventure.

*Just make sure to label and date your products very carefully and keep out of reach of small children.

Below is a list of supplies and ingredients that you will need to keep on hand or purchase ahead of time depending upon what you will be making for the day. Just remember that it will take several days to have supplies shipped to you. So there is a bit of planning involved in making salves and ointments. You will have to have some patience when going into this endeavor but the rewards are really worth it!

Supplies & Ingredients

- Isopropyl Alcohol at least 90%
- Olive Oil
- Coconut Oil
- Almond Oil
- Apricot Oil
- Jojoba Oil
- Sesame Oil
- Sunflower Oil
- Rice Bran Oil
- Avocado Oil
- Grape Seed Oil
- Emu Oil or Blue Emu (This make the cannabis absorb into the skin better)

- Aloe Vera Gel
- Beeswax
- Vegetable wax like, Candelilla or Carnauba
- Shea Butter
- Essential Oils
  - Rosemary
  - Lavender
  - Orange
  - Lemon
  - Calendula
  - Cinnamon
  - Clove
  - Myrrh
  - Black Pepper
  - Cumin
  - Coriander
- Cocoa Butter
- Mango Butter
- Healing Flowers like Calendula, etc
- Alcohol Tinctures
  - Arnica Montana
  - Calendula
  - St. Johns Wort
  - Lavender
  - Magnesium Chloride Oil (for severe pain or gout)

Remember you will not use all of these ingredients but you will use some of them so make sure that you have at least one oil you like working with, a few essential oils that you like, and know ahead of time if you are making an ointment, salve, or tincture. You will save a lot of time and money if you start small and then work up to a master mixologist!

Now it looks like you are getting ready to start on your endeavor! Just remember you can't fail. You can just improve on what you are doing! Most of all be careful and be cautious at all times. You do not want to burn yourself or destroy your kitchen supplies. Keep yourself aware and alert for this entire process.

Making salves and ointments is an art form so make sure you also use your creative juices when thinking of what you will be using the ointment for and how you want it to smell and look like. Once you get the basic steps down you can then start to be creative and cater to specific ailments that you or your friends have and make ointments, salves, and tinctures that are both healing and have great aromatherapy qualities!

Kitchen Notes

Kitchen Notes

Types of Topical Cannabis Products

Extraction

There are many ways that you can extract the cannabinoids from the plant. There are also many avenues in which to use the extracted cannabis either in creams, salves, ointments, or tinctures. We will go over tinctures first and then move on to cannabis oils, salves, and ointments.

Types of Cannabis

First of all let's make sure that you are using the correct cannabis product for making ointments, salves, and tinctures. There are two types of cannabis strains. One is Indica and one is Sativa.

It is best to use a cannabis plant that is mostly Indica based because it will help with physical symptoms better than Sativa. Indica helps to reduce pain, relax muscles, and reduce inflammation. Indica tends to have higher concentrations of CBD (cannabinoids or THC) so it is preferred more for inhaling or ingesting for medicinal purposes, but if you are unsure what strain you have then experiment with what you have or ask your doctor who prescribed the medicinal cannabis for you. It never hurts to try something new. They only difference will be the potency of the product but the product will still be good and useful for many different ailments and skin diseases.

So make sure that you check with your doctor or dispensary to see what type of plant you are using or which type of plant is in the product you are purchasing.

Tinctures

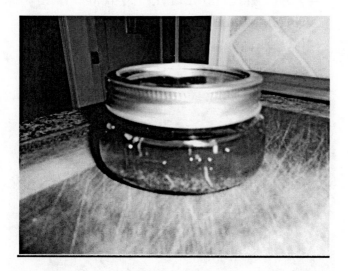

REMEMBER THESE ARE NON EDIBLE TINCTURES!

Tinctures are perfect for using on your sore spastic muscles or if you have one of the many debilitating arthritic diseases.

One method of extracting the THC from the cannabis is called, cold extraction. This is one of the easiest ways to make a healing cannabis product but it does take more time to extract the cannabinoids because cold extraction is a slower process.

1. You can do this by measuring 1 oz (28 grams) of cannabis to 1 pint of **rubbing** alcohol or another easy way to measure is to use any type of glass jar and fill it 25% full of dry crushed cannabis and 3-4 parts of rubbing alcohol.

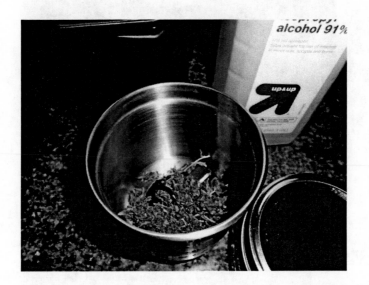

2. Start with ground cold cannabis and add it to the **rubbing** alcohol in a large glass jar. **Do not use plastic bottles for this process!**

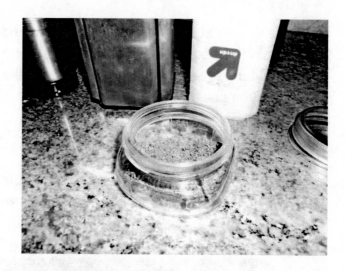

3. Shake the mixture for 5 minutes and then put in a dark shady area for 2-3 weeks.

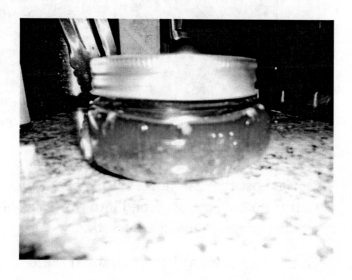

4. After several weeks take the mixture and strain it through cheesecloth, coffee filters, or nylons several different times to make sure that you get the cannabis powder removed. I personally used cheesecloth but it is entirely up to you and what supplies that you have.

5. You can also save the filtered cannabis in the cheesecloth to rub on sore muscles for relief from pain.

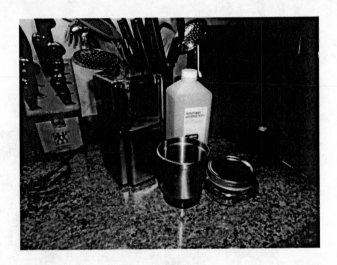

*It is also best to wear gloves during both processes so that it doesn't get absorbed into the skin while straining it through the cheesecloth.

Once the cannabis has been extracted the tinctures can be kept in the freezer or refrigerator so that they will last longer.

There are over 100 types of arthritis out there but the one thing that all of these types of arthritis have in common is that there is a constant destruction of the cartilage in the body and joint tissue loss. By using the cannabis infused rubbing alcohol on your arthritic hands, feet, knees, etc, you can help ease the pain and suffering along with helping to reduce the deteriorating cartilage in the joints. **Be aware that the green color of the rubbing alcohol may stain your clothing so wear something that you don't mind if you ruin.**

*ALSO BEWARE THAT ISOPROPYL ALCOHOL IS HIGHLY FLAMMABLE SO KEEP FROM HEAT, SPARK, ELETRICAL, OR FIRES! I STORE THE JARS IN A DARK CLOSET AWAY FROM ANYTHING FLAMMABLE.

<u>Please refer to my first book Treating Holistically with Cannabis Updated and Expanded for more information on tinctures that you can ingest.</u>

After Soaking for One Week

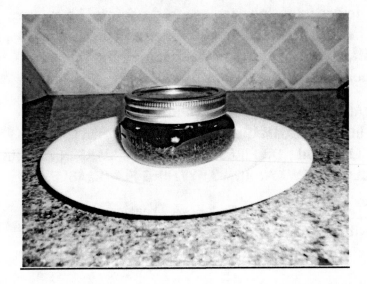

Notes

Notes

Cannabis Oils

Cannabis oil can be made from many different types of oils and in several different ways. It is important that you experiment with what types of oils you like and what process you like the best.

One of the best oils to use is emu but it is difficult to find and expensive, but there are other oils out there that are just as good like, almond, apricot, sunflower, calendula, olive, rice bran, avocado, grape seed, olive, and coconut. It is best to stick with just one type oil for each batch (until you are more experienced at mixing the different consistencies and absorption rates of oils) and then add your essential oils at the end of the process to give your oil different healing qualities and scents. I prefer to use coconut oil because it has the highest fat content of any oil, which makes it easier to be absorbed into the skin and better in the extraction of cannabis process. Cannabis oil can be made into a great salve by adding beeswax along with different essential oils.

Make sure that when you are looking for your coconut oils that you are purchasing organic virgin cold pressed oil. You might as well use the best on your skin. Just remember, your skin care products are only as good as the ingredients that you use to create them!

Cold Extraction

1. Take a jar and add enough cannabis to fill it ¼ of the way and then fill the rest with your favorite oil.
2. Make sure that you shake the mixture <u>daily</u> and store in a dark place for a month or so.
3. Once you have done this then it is ready to filter through cheesecloth and then it's ready for use.
4. Again save the filtered particles with the cheesecloth and you can use it as a rub or poultice.

*I would not recommend using hemp oil because it has been known to not emulsify as well as coconut oil with cannabis and sometimes gives you a lumpy product but it is entirely up to your preference.

Warm Extraction

1. 2 cups organic cold pressed coconut oil.

2. Heat oven to 200 degrees and crush 2 cups of cannabis and place in a baking dish and bake for 10 minutes. If your cannabis is really dry you may not need to do this process.
3. Grind up the cannabis into a smooth powder with a coffee grinder or a dry mix vita mixer.
4. Place the cannabis into the coconut oil, stir gently, and simmer on the lowest setting on your stove for about 1-2 hours. You can also use a crock pot if you would like. It's really up to you.
5. Strain with cheesecloth, coffee filter, nylons (make sure they are new because of contamination), or a really fine mesh strainer. If there are too many chunks left in the mixture you can restrain the mixture again until you have no debris left in the oil.

The above recipe works well, but if you want a more precise recipe mixture then use the information below.

Here are some measuring amounts that I use as guidelines when making cannabis oil but there are different measurements out there and you will have to experiment to see what works for you.

*For 14-16 oz of coconut oil I use anywhere from 25 grams to 35 grams of cannabis. It will depend on the quality of the cannabis and the potency you are looking for. Remember 28 grams equals 1 oz.

I wanted to note that it is not always necessary to cook the cannabis first in the oven before you mix it with the coconut oil (or other oils). It will depend on how dry your product is but the process will work just as well if you do not cook it first. I also like to grind up my cannabis into a fine powder when I am making my cannabis oil. I find that it is better to use the ratio of approximately 28-35 grams of cannabis to 14 oz of coconut oil.

Another Warm Cooking Method

1. Another way to make cannabis oil is to start with a large canning pan and some canning jars.
2. Next take and fill the jars ¾ of the way with cannabis leaves and buds and then the rest of the jar with the oil of your choice.
3. Make sure to put the lids on the jars tight so that water will not seep through the lids.
4. Next put enough water in the pan so that the water sits right below the neck of the jars.
5. You will need to use extra lids to set the jars on in the pan because they should not be set directly on the bottom of the pan.
6. Stir the mixture a couple of times an hour. You will cook this mixture for 6-8 hours.

7. Make sure to also keep an eye on the water in the pan because it will evaporate and you will need to add more during this long process.

8. Now take the mixture and strain it with cheesecloth or if you have an extra pair of nylons you could use them and then put the mixture back into the jars and refrigerate. Do Not Freeze this mixture.

Easy Warm Cannabis Oil Recipe

(This is the one I use)

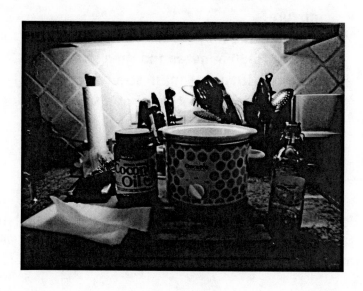

1. 14-16 oz of Coconut Oil
2. 25-35 Grams of Cannabis
3. Grind up the cannabis into a fine powder with a coffee grinder.
4. Measure out 14-16 oz of coconut oil and place into a crock pot that is on low or better yet on warm if your crock pot has that setting.
5. Sift the finely ground cannabis and then add to the oil.
6. Cook the mixture for anywhere from 1-2 hours. If your crock pot only has a low heating setting than I would go for the 1 hour, but if you have a crock pot with a warm setting I would go 1 ½ to 2 hours. Make sure that you check on it every half an hour to make sure that it is not burning. Each crock pot and each stove is different so it is best to err on the side of caution. You don't want to burn the mixture.
7. Now that the mixture is strained let it cool for around 15-30 minutes and then strain the mixture with a fine mesh strainer or cheesecloth. I sometimes put a small piece of cheesecloth in the bottom of the fine mesh strainer to give it an extra straining.
8. Now your product is ready for mixing with essential oils, beeswax, Shea butter, etc.

*Please note that you can also use the cannabis oil as an ingredient in your medibles BEFORE YOU ADD THE SHEA BUTTER, ESSENTIAL OILS, BEEWAX, ETC!!!!!!

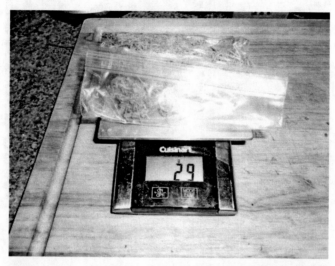

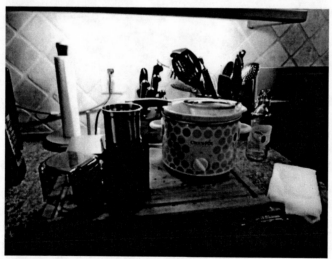

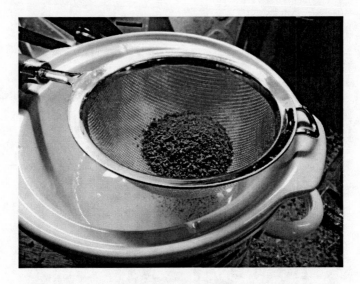

Coconut Oil and ground up cannabis

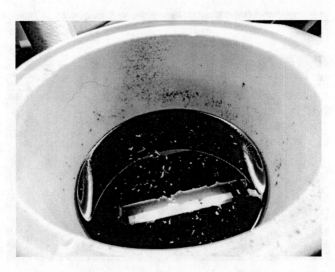

After about 1 hour of cooking

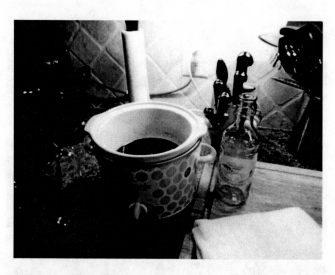

*You can also make a half batch if you just want to have a smaller amount around. Make sure that you use your product soon instead of leaving it around the house because it will lose its potency within six months to a year. You can also keep it in the refrigerator to give the product a longer shelf life.

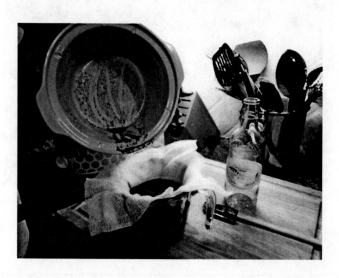

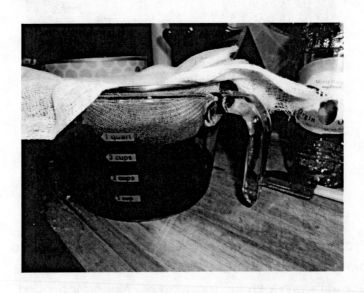

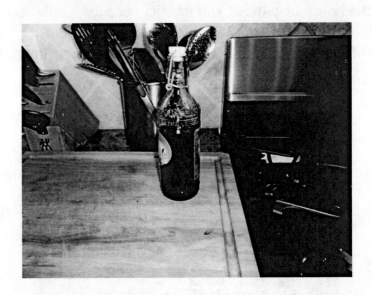

Now you will want to save the strained material! I have seen this made into some cleaver items.

1. Save for a poultice and as a rub for sore muscles.
2. Mix with a bit of coconut oil and reheat on stove on low heat and then add chocolate, nuts, and berries and make into a candy bar.
3. Mix with a bit of coconut oil and salt or sugar and make a body scrub.

Please refer to my first book Treating Holistically with Cannabis Updated and Expanded for more information on cannabis oil recipes that you can ingest. The above oil can be used in recipes or used with other ingredients as a salve or ointment! Make sure you label your medicine so that you know what you have!!!!

Body Scrub

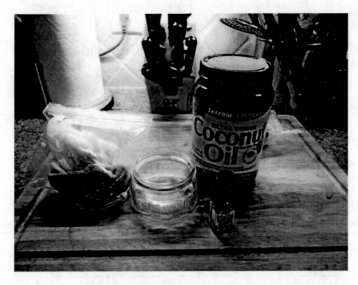

Use Coconut Oil or Olive Oil

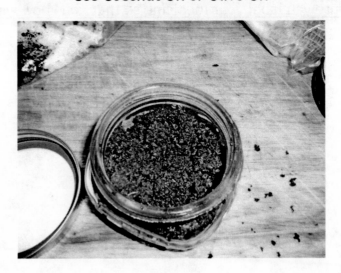

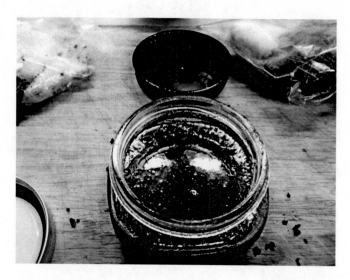

Cover Cannabis with Your Preferred Oil

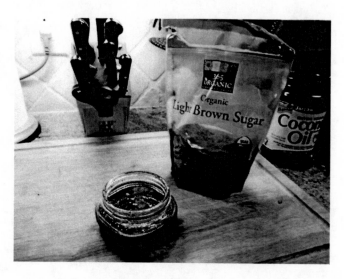

Brown Sugar Added To Scrub

Notes

Notes

Notes

Ointments

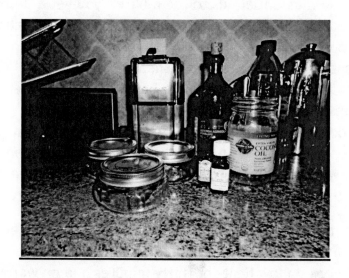

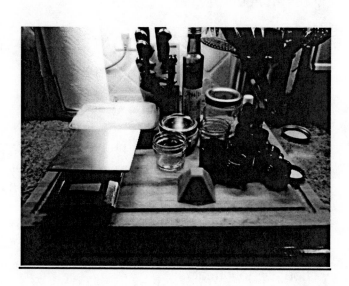

Ointments are another great way for you to get your topical cannabis. Ointments are more nourishing to your body and make your skin really soft plus once you add essential oils to the mixture you get a better product that has a great scent and has better healing properties. Shea butter ointments will be runny in consistency compared to a Shea butter salve or cannabis oil salve. The more beeswax you use the harder the product will be. If you want a thicker product than use more beeswax in the recipe, but then you will end up with a salve. It's really depends on what you want. You can also store your ointments in the refrigerator, which will make them thicker.

To make an ointment you will need a double boiler or a crock pot (if you use a crock pot you will need to cook on low heat for thirty minutes and on warm setting for an hour).

Long Method for Ointment

1. This is the best ratio if you have large leaves and your cannabis is not ground up fine yet: Cannabis 25% to 75% of Shea butter. I use 8 oz of Shea butter to 1/2 oz (14 grams) of cannabis.
2. Heat it up in a double boiler for around an hour on low heat.

3. Make sure that your cannabis is completely dried and chopped up into small pieces (not super fine).
4. Make sure that the Shea butter is completely melted and kept stirring the mixture. You will need to do this for 1 hour to infuse the Shea butter with the cannabis.
5. Once this is done you will need to store the mixture for a couple of months.
6. After that you will need to reheat the mixture and add a small amount of beeswax to the mixture to give the ointment the right consistency. You will know the right consistency when you test the ointment to see if it thickens up when cooled. It will depend on what you like best. If you would like more of a lotion consistency then you can add less beeswax and add a bit of aloe vera gel to the mixture.
7. After that you will need to strain the mixture and store in smaller jars in the refrigerator.

*You can also use Cocoa Butter instead of Shea Butter. They are very similar but from different plants.

Shea Butter comes from the seed of the Shea tree, which is from Africa. Shea Butter has a creamy soft texture and smells nuttier than Cocoa Butter.

Cocoa Butter comes from the cocoa bean and has a rich chocolaty smell and is not as creamy and soft.

They are both great choices it really just depends on what you have on hand and what your preferences are. I love them both!

Short Method for Ointment

This is my favorite method!

1. 7 oz of Shea butter
2. 1 oz of Coconut oil
3. 1 oz of Avocado oil
4. 25 grams of cannabis
5. Add your mixture to a double boiler or a crock pot and heat mixture until it is all melted together. Make sure to keep an eye on the mixture and stir every once in a while. Cook for around an hour in a crock pot or 2 hours on with a double boiler. I prefer a double boiler because it doesn't get as hot and you can monitor it better.
6. Let cool for around one hour
7. Strain and then add your essential oils (around 20 droplets) and if it appears too thick you can add a bit of almond oil if you would like. It is up to your preference on what consistency you would like.
8. You can store your medicine in the refrigerator but just remember that the

consistency will be different when you leave it in the refrigerator compared to leaving it in the cupboard. If you know that you want to use your medicine make sure to take it out of the refrigerator ahead of time so that it will give it some time to be malleable. Just remember to not freeze the mixture.

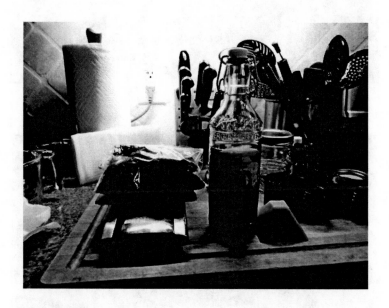

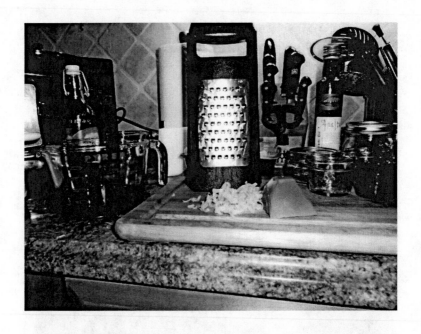

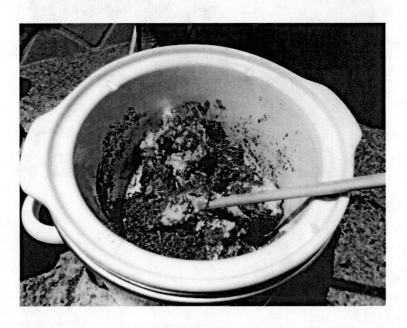

*Make sure when you add all of the ingredients together that you are stirring constantly until it turns to a liquid and so that it does not burn. Crock pot method.

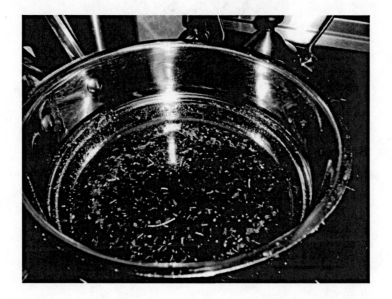

Double Boiler Method

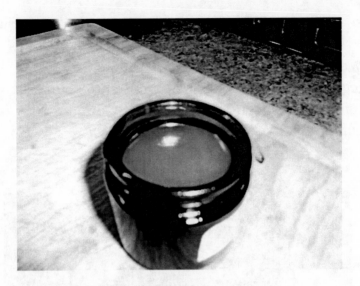

Finished Ointment

As you can see the consistency is thinner than the salves or coconut oil and beeswax product, again you can store it in the refrigerator to make a thicker product.

Notes

Notes

Salves

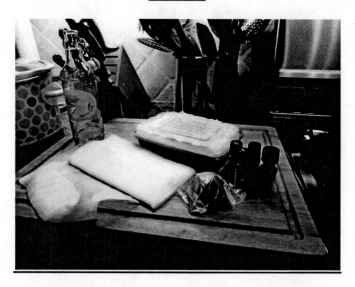

To make a salve you will need a double boiler or a crock pot (if you use a crock pot you will need to cook on low heat for thirty minutes and if your crock pot has a warm setting let it cook for one hour):

1. Use this ratio: 25% cannabis to 50% Shea butter and 25 % beeswax. (The salve will have much more beeswax than the ointment).
2. Heat the beeswax, cocoa butter, and cannabis until melted about 45-60 minutes. Make sure to either use beeswax pellets or grate the beeswax first. *Make sure you use a grater that you don't mind getting wax all over because it is difficult to clean. I think if you chop the beeswax into small pieces it works just as well.

3. Again you will need to let the salve sit for a couple months.
4. After it has sat for two months then reheat mixture and then filter the mixture through cheesecloth.
5. Now add to your favorite jars with your favorite essential oils.

Another easy way to make salve is to start with the cannabis oil recipe

1. 5 oz of cannabis oil that you already made.
2. Then mix in 1 oz of grated beeswax.
3. Heat this slowly on the stove for 15 minutes or until melted.
4. Before your mixture cools add 1 vitamin E capsule to the mixture and you are done! Some people like the vitamin E capsule and some don't it because it makes the mixture a bit on the oily side but it is really up to you. I would add some essential oils also at this point.

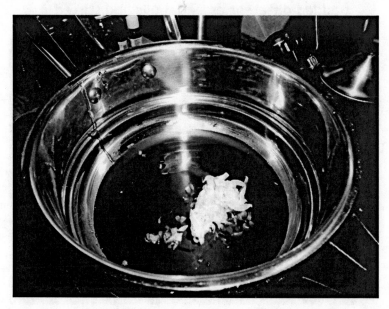

Grated Beeswax and Cannabis Oil

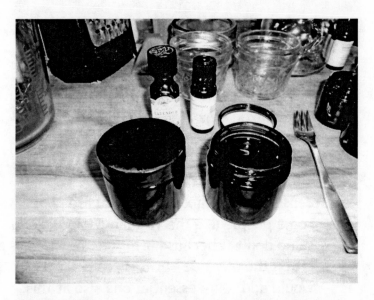

I added the cannabis coconut oil to jars and then
added different essential oils and stirred

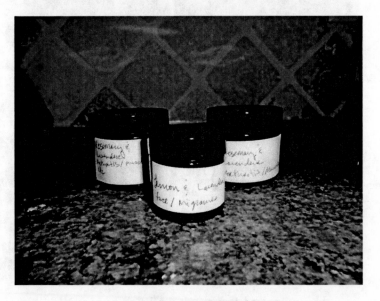

Finished Product

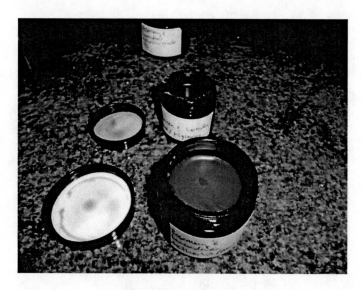

Finished Consistency

There are also a couple of other different waxes that you could use instead of beeswax (which comes in white and yellow: bleached and unbleached. Best to use unbleached) and they are made of vegetables. They are carnauba and candelilla wax. If you are going to use candelilla wax it's made from the leaves of a shrub native to Mexico and is slightly harder than beeswax so you will need to use less in the recipes. Carnauba is a wax made from a Brazilian Palm. I always prefer to use beeswax but it is really up to your preference.

A good measure is 20% beeswax to 80% cannabis oil.

*I WOULD NOT RECOMMEND USING ANY OF THESE PRODUCTS AROUND YOUR EYES BECAUSE IT WILL MAKE THE EYES APPEAR TO BE STONED, RED AND GLOSSY FOR UP TO 8 HRS.

Easy Salve Method

1. 4 oz of Shea butter
2. 25-28 grams of cannabis (ground up fine)
3. 2 oz of beeswax
4. In a double boiler heat the mixture together on low. Keep stirring until mixture is well mixed together. Cook mixture for around 2 hours and occasionally stir the mixture so that it does not burn on the bottom on the pan. *It works best to add a couple tablespoons of coconut oil to the bottom of the pan at first because the Shea butter and the beeswax are really thick.
5. Let mixture cool for around 30 minutes and then use cheese cloth and a strainer to strain mixture. Now place the mixture into you containers and then add the type of essential oils that you would like to the mixture. I add about 10 drops per every 2 oz of product but it will be up to your preference.

6. Let set for a couple of hours and refrigerate if you are not going to use right away.

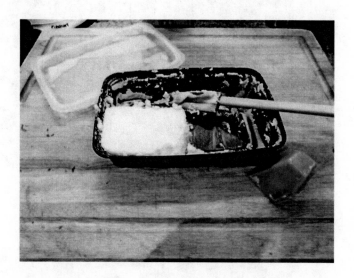

Shea butter and beeswax

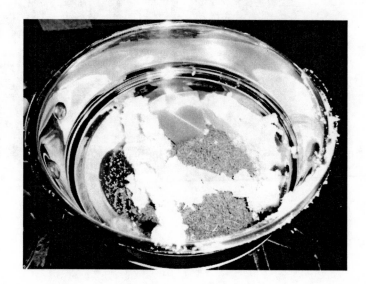

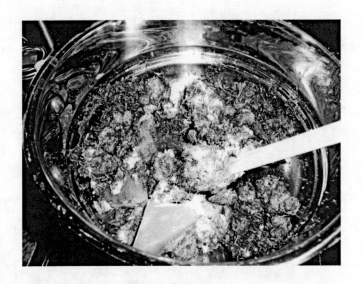

Keep Stirring

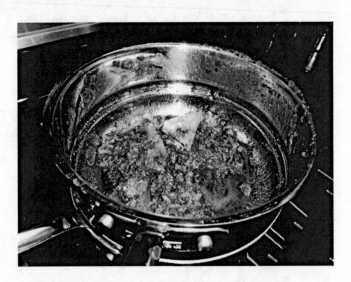

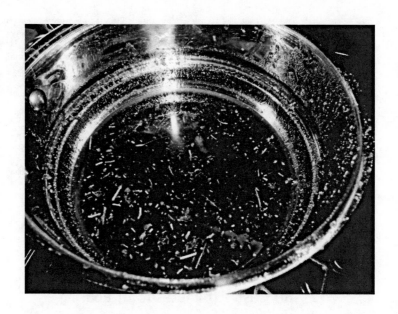

Double Boiler Method

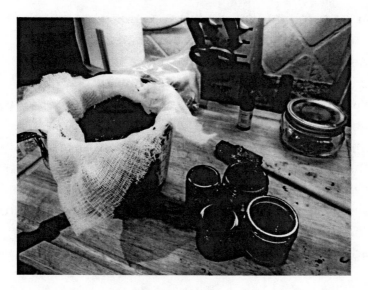

Straining Cannabis

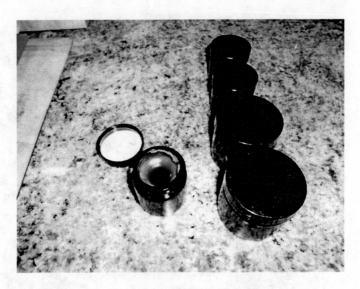

Just 15 minutes After Pouring

Make sure that you move fast at this point since the salves have more beeswax in the mixture, it gets thicker quicker! You will have to add the essential oils quickly and make sure that you stir between each pour because the mixture will start to set very quickly and you want to make sure that your whole mixture has the same amount of essential oils throughout. Again you can store these in the refrigerator to prolong their life, but just remember since there is more beeswax in this recipe make sure to take the salve out of the refrigerator well in advanced of wanting to use the product.

Notes

Notes

ESSENTIAL OILS

As you probably already know essential oils are very beneficial to you and your health, especially when mixed with cannabis. Essential oils are not really oils at all. Essential oils are really just a super concentration of plant or flower extracts. They should not be used directly on the skin but mixed with a carrier oil such as coconut or olive oil. Essential oils can last anywhere up to 10 years, so it may seem expensive at first but look at how many years of use you will get. Store them in a dark place out of sunlight.

Cannabis and many essential oils have terpenes, which alter sensitivity, balance, and pain within the body. There are over 100 terpenes in cannabis. Terpenes in cannabis are found in the resin so when cannabis is heated up (as in making salves and ointments) you will have many terpenes in your salves and when you mix them with the terpenes that are in essential oils you will have so much more power!

It is important when you are making you salves and ointments to remember what ailment you are making the salve for like, acne, arthritis, sore muscles, insect bites, eczema, migraines, chapped skin, etc. Make small batches so that you can add the appropriate essential oil to your mixture to give your salves an extra boost to help what ails you! Adding essential oils to your mixtures is really where your salves will shine.

You will need to experiment and go by the list below as a guide for your ailments. You can't really mess up as long as you have a great salve or ointment base to start with. So start with the cannabis oil, salve, and ointment recipes in the book first and then build your own potion with the essential oils below. You can also just use the oils, ointments, and salves without essential oils, but I like to give my salves character plus I love the added benefits of essential oils.

Let's start with rosemary oil. Rosemary oil is great for stimulating your circulation due to ailments such as arthritis, gout, muscle cramping, and rheumatism. Rosemary is also great to combat acne so adding it to your cannabis salves will be really beneficial. Rosemary also has many terperens which help to restore memory loss. This is a great oil to add to any of you salves or ointments.

Cinnamon essential oil is great for arthritis, low blood pressure, and exhaustion. It has a really nice smell but make sure to not use this near or around the face!

Lavender oil is used in so many things in our everyday life. Lavender oil has stress healing qualities along with physical ailments like burns, boils, cuts, cystitis, eczema, insect bites, muscle aches, strains, sprains, headaches, migraines, dermatitis, itching, scars, sores, stress, and wounds. This is one of the best essential oils that you can add to you salves and if you add rosemary along with it you will have one powerful salve!

Cedarwood is great for acne, arthritis, dermatitis, and stress. It has an earthy smell that is really nice.

Clove oil is great for arthritis, asthma, sprains, and strains. Canella oil (cinnamon) can be mixed with clove oil for an extra healing process.

Lemon oil is great for athlete's feet, dull skin, oily skin, varicose veins, warts, and has anti-cancer properties. Lemon or any citrus oil is extremely high is terpenes!

Myrrh oil is good for athlete's feet, itchy skin and chapped skin.

Juniper oil is used for acne, cellulites, gout, and for toxin buildup. You could use just this oil for a gout remedy! Great stuff!

Basil oil is good for gout, insect bites, muscle aches, and rheumatism. This is yet awesome oil for gout! It appears that our country has an excess of patients with gout. It would be too simple to try to make a salve with cannabis and basil or juniper oil!

Eucalyptus oil is great for arthritis and poor circulation. This is a bit strong so make sure you do not get this in your eyes or anywhere around your face.

Cumin oil is great for people with poor circulation, low blood pressure, and toxin buildup.

Coriander oil is great for aches, arthritis, gout, and rheumatism.

Black pepper oil is good for aching muscles, arthritis, muscle cramps, and poor circulation. Black pepper also has many terpenes that are good as an analgesic and helps reduce inflammation.

Sage oil can be mixed with lavender oil and rosemary oil to make a great salve that heals and restores your energy in the body.

There are many more essential oils out there that you can experiment with but these are some of my favorites that I use in my salves and ointments. Try your own mixtures and see how they work for you. It's a great way to get more power into your salves and ointments.

Please remember to keep all of your essential oils and medicines out of reach from little hands.

BENEFITS OF OILS

Using the right oils on your skin is really important. If you want to add a bit of these oils to your salves or ointments at the end of the process or at the same time that you add your other essential oils you will have some of the most beneficial salves on the planet! Make sure to not add too much but just a 1/8 of a cup to your whole batch will be really beneficial to your skin. You may want to experiment with the texture that you like best but it is ok to experiment. Making salves and ointments is supposed to be fun! I still prefer to use coconut oil in most of my recipes but you will find what you like the best.

I wanted to go over some of the best ones to use on your skin or hair.

Almond oil is beneficial because it is easily absorbed into the skin and many vitamins like A, B1, B2, B6, and E. Almond oil helps with relieving dry itchy skin and also helps to nourish your hair.

Apricot oil also absorbs into the skin very easily and has vitamins A, D, and E and is good for inflammation and itchy skin.

Avocado oil is good for sun damaged and aging skin. Avocado oil has vitamins A, D, E, B1, B2, and E.

Grape seed oil is a wonderful lightweight oil that is easily absorbed into the skin.

Jojoba oil is not really an oil at all but a liquid wax. Jojoba helps with acne, inflammation, and on aging skin.

Olive oil has great properties and it needs to be purchased cold pressed. Olive oil resembles your skin the best. Olive oil forms a protective layer on your skin.

Sesame oil is one of the most nutritional oils for your skin. Sesame oil has vitamins E, B, and A. Sesame oil has a special ingredient called sesamol that helps with wrinkles.

Walnut oil has many great qualities for your skin and hair. Walnut oil is easily absorbed into the skin and has a mild astringent quality that helps gives your skin antibacterial properties.

TESTIMONIALS

I HAVE HAD A BAD BACK FOR YEARS! NOTHING SEEMED TO HELP UNTIL I TRIED CANNABIS SALVES. I ALMOST COULDN'T BELIEVE IT. WITHIN A COUPLE OF DAYS OF APPLICATION I FELT LIKE I WAS HEALED! WHAT A GREAT PRODUCT!

MICHAEL SHORES

AFTER DRIVING ON A LONG TRIP I ARRIVED WITH A VERY BAD HEADACHE AND A REALLY SORE NECK. I HAD REMEMBERED THAT I HAD SOME CANNABIS OINTMENT IN MY BAG. I WAS SO RELIEVED THAT I HAD IT WITH ME. I IMMEDIATELY PUT SOME CANNABIS OINTMENT ON MY NECK AND WITHIN AN HOUR THE PAIN WAS ALMOST GONE. I CONTINUED TO APPLY THE CANNABIS OINTMENT FOR A COUPLE OF DAYS UNTIL IT WAS COMPLETELY GONE. I AM SO HAPPY THAT I HAD SOME CANNABIS OINTMENT WITH ME.

SORE SAM

FOR YEARS I HAVE HAD SUN DAMAGE ON MY SHOULDERS AND I WANTED TO SEE IF CANNABIS SALVE WOULD HELP BECAUSE I HEARD THAT IT CAN HELP WITH BURNS AND SKIN DISCOLORATION. I DECIDED THAT I WOULD TRY THE CANNABIS SALVE TO SEE WHAT WOULD HAPPEN. WITHIN A WEEK I COULD SEE A HUGE DIFFERENCE. I WAS AMAZED. I WILL KEEP USING THIS PRODUCT FOR AS LONG AS I CAN!

SUN~BURNT CITIZEN

FEELINGS, AFFECTS, & DOSAGE LOG

*IT IS IMPORTANT TO WRITE DOWN THE AFFECTS AND THE DOSAGE OF WHAT YOU HAVE USED! YOU MAY EVEN FIND THAT YOU HAVE YOUR OWN RECIPES YOU WANT TO WRITE DOWN AND REMEMBER! PLEASE BE CAUTIOUS AND START OUT WITH SMALL DOSAGES!

DOSAGE:_____

_____

AFFECTS:_____

_____

PRODUCT:_____

_____

_____

DOSAGE:_____

_____

AFFECTS:_____

_____

PRODUCT:_____

_____

DOSAGE:_____

_____

AFFECTS:_____

PRODUCT:_____

DOSAGE:_____

AFFECTS:_____

PRODUCT:_____

DOSAGE:_____

AFFECTS:_____

PRODUCT:_____

DOSAGE:_____

AFFECTS:_____
PRODUCT:_____

DOSAGE:_____

_____

AFFECTS:_____

_____

PRODUCT:_____

_____

DOSAGE:_____

_____

AFFECTS:_____

_____

PRODUCT:_____

_____

DOSAGE:_____

_____

AFFECTSS:_____

_____

PRODUCT:_____

_____

_____

DOSAGE:_____

_____

AFFECTS:_____

_____

PRODUCT:_____

_____

DOSAGE:_____

_____

AFFECTS:_____

_____

PRODUCT:_____

_____

DOSAGE:_____

_____

AFFECTS:_____

_____

PRODUCT:_____

_____

DOSAGE:_____

_____

_____

AFFECTS:_____

_____

PRODUCT:_____

DOSAGE:_____

AFFFECTS:_____

PRODUCT:_____

DOSAGE:_____

AFFECTS:_____

PRODUCT:_____

DOSAGE:_____

AFFECTS:_____

PRODUCT:_____

RECIPES NOTES:

_____

_____

_____

_____

_____

_____

_____

_____

_____

_____

_____

_____

_____

_____

_____

_____

_____

_____

_____

ABOUT THE AUTHOR:

Bachelors of Science in Physical Anthropology, Minor in Business, and Culinary Arts Degree.

Advocate for organic, vegetarian, vegan, raw food diets, writing, yoga, biking, and running! Interested in making the world a better place through diet, nutrition, and natural healing!

For more information on how to order books, original articles, updates on future projects go to www.TreatingHolisticallywithCannabis.com

I hope you enjoy my cannabis recipes and insights!

I hope that they help with all of your ailments!

If you have any suggestions, comments, or corrections please feel free to email me at sunnycabanapublishing@gmail.com or TreatingHolisticallyCannabis@gmail.com

Follow our blog at:
TreatingHolisticallywithCannabis.blogspot.com

Follow us on facebook at:
facebook.com/sunnycabanapublishing

*Please make sure that you label all of your medicines and keep them far away from small hands.

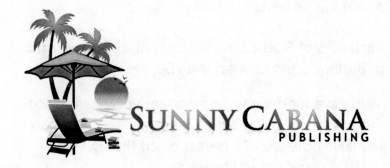

SUNNY CABANA
PUBLISHING

CHECK OUT MY FIRST BOOK

$9.99

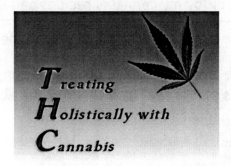

*T*reating
*H*olistically with
*C*annabis

Vegetarian medical marijuana recipes, tinctures,
& health benefits for what ails you!

UPDATED & EXPANDED

Marie J. Burke

Helpful Magazines

(Some of these are online magazines)

High Times Magazine

Treating Yourself: The Alternative Medicine Journal

Cannabis Culture Magazine

Skunk Magazine

Kush Magazine

420 Magazine

Helpful Websites

www.norml.org

www.medicalmarijuana.org

www.kingstoncompassion.org

www.medcannaccess.ca

www.medicalmarijuanaofamerica.com

www.peopleadvocatingcannabiseducation.org

www.docgreens.org

www.apothecanna.com

www.theweedtour.com

www.cremedecanna.com

www.grasscity.com

www.GrowKind.com

www.weedtracker.com

www.rollitup.com

www.weedmaps.com

www.Amazon.com

www.tetralabs.com

*Please check your area to make sure it is LEGAL to have medical cannabis in your possession!

Index

CPSIA information can be obtained at www.ICGtesting.com
Printed in the USA
LVOW08s1950020414

380037LV00001B/163/P